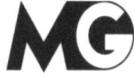

MG

Notice

The contents of this book or guide are only given as a form of advice and suggestions. If you suffer from any health issues, discuss this book and its contents with your health professional before using it. The author and publisher assume no responsibility or liability for any errors or omissions in the content of this book and do not provide medical advice.

Published by MassoGuide

www.massoguide.com

ISBN : 978-1-7778345-9-3

First edition - Paper - 2021

Vous retrouverez dans ce livre

Introduction

We all commonly develop muscle tension or «knots» in our bodies. It is part of our shared reality as humans. They bother us, irritate us and annoy us with their presence.

These situations are often described to massage therapists by their clients: neck tension, lower back tenderness, tender knee, and even more! Even if massage can help lessen the effects of the tensions, it is pretty common for them to come back if the reasons for their presence are not corrected. However, it is possible to help yourself in the meantime with some well-targeted self-massage techniques.

Self-massage allows you to control your tensions, reduce their effects, and remove them. My objective with this guide is to offer you the same advice that I present to my clients. These will help you target precisely the correct muscles and show you how to relax them. This book series uses different tools and methods that complement each other.

The ball, the foam roller, the massage gun, and the stretching exercises offer various options to help you. All of them are easily accessible to you and require very little time to learn and do. I offer you this book to help you find those annoying sore spots that hassle you so that you can relax them efficiently.

Enjoy.

Terms glossary

Micromovements:

Very small back and forth movements.

Microrotations:

Very small rotations.

Massage:

To use the massage gun on a muscle or an area of your body.

Soreness:

The different sensations you feel when you self-massage, and there is some discomfort.

Pressure:

Refers to the level of depth that is reached when massaging a muscle. You will generally find the following levels: superficial, medium et deep.

Pain:

Refers to any soreness that has reached the pain threshold.

Health problem:

Any pathology or health issue.

How to use this book

Movements

You should follow the instructions on the different illustrations in order to know which area you should massage. When you use a massage gun, you should, most of the time, hold it with the hand from the opposite side to the one you wish to massage.

Be sure to take the time that's necessary to do each movement thoroughly. If you omit parts of the muscle, you will not be relaxing it to its fullest extent.

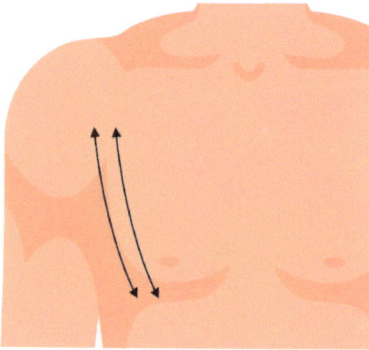

Rotations allow you to relax an area with precision.

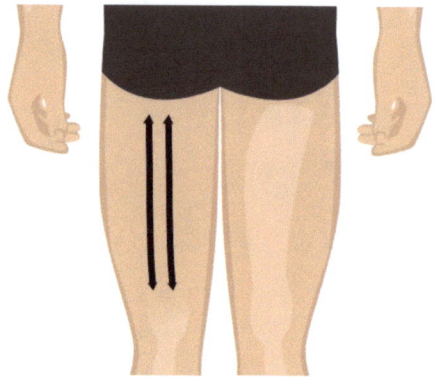

Lines allow you to relax an area or the totality of a muscle.

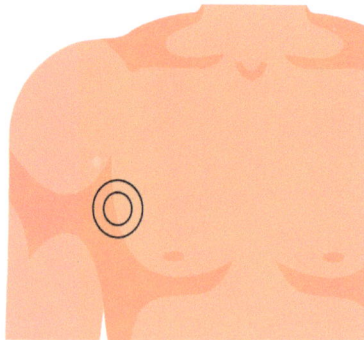

Pressure points allow you to relax slowly the deepest of tensions.

Pressure

To correctly rate the level of soreness felt and that you should look at reaching to obtain an effective tension release, follow this rule that we also use during a massage using zero to ten: if zero equals no soreness and ten equals actual pain, the desired level in self-massage is generally between 3 and 5.

This way, you get to feel the muscle release while staying away from the dangerous pain threshold. It also helps you assess your massage's effectiveness and notice how the soreness level evolves. You can work at increasing it or at lowering it.

Soreness level	Quantity	Description
Almost nothing	0 to 3	You feel nothing at all or almost nothing.
A little	3 to 5	Relaxes you, allows you to slowly begin to self-massage and explore your body to find the tensed areas. It also allows to massage very sore areas slowly, layer by layer.
Average	5 to 6	Good pressure. Remember to adjust if the area is sore. The ideal level for daily muscle tension.
High	7 to 8	Soreness that is at a high level and approaching the limit.
Very high	8 to 10	Very high level of soreness you will not find comfortable. It is also at 10 that the pain level begins, which must not be reached.

During a self-massage, always aim for a soreness level between 3 to 5 out of 10.

Breathing

Make sure to keep breathing while you self-massage: you will prevent your muscle from relaxing if the soreness level becomes so intense that you stop breathing.

Keep an eye on your breathing: a slow exhale that is also deep and controlled is ideal. You do not have to worry about inhaling as it will adjust itself on its own if you exhale slowly.

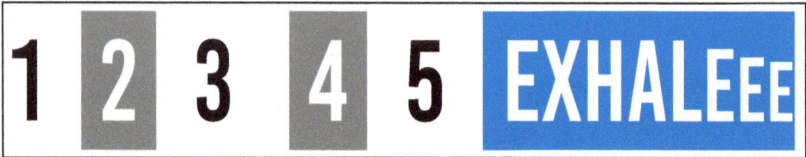

1 2 3 4 5 EXHALEEE

Be sure to keep your hand relaxed while you are self-massaging. Same thing if you are using a massage gun. It is useless to relax an area while you tensed up another one.

Duration

Very little time is needed to relax a muscle. When you self-massage, the minimum recommended duration is of 90 seconds per area or per muscle. The gun allows you to cover a large area easily and quickly.

The objective is to reduce your tensions, and for this purpose, you need to take the time it takes. However, there are limits, and after a certain amount of time, you will not see any more results. In some cases, if you do not respect the limits, continuing can even become problematic and become unhealthy.

Always keep in mind the 90 seconds golden rule and keep on respecting the other limits, especially the depth and pressure limits, to ensure you achieve an efficient and safe relaxing of your muscles. However, be careful not to limit yourself to this tool as the gun is not a complete solution, and in some areas, it might not be the best tool to meet all your needs.

You can do an exercise two or three times a week as it seems to fit most people's needs. However, if you are physically active, you might have to increase the number of weekly repetitions to achieve the same result.

90 seconds
minimum

The sore areas

Zones and soreness

Massage the selected muscles according to the highlighted zone.

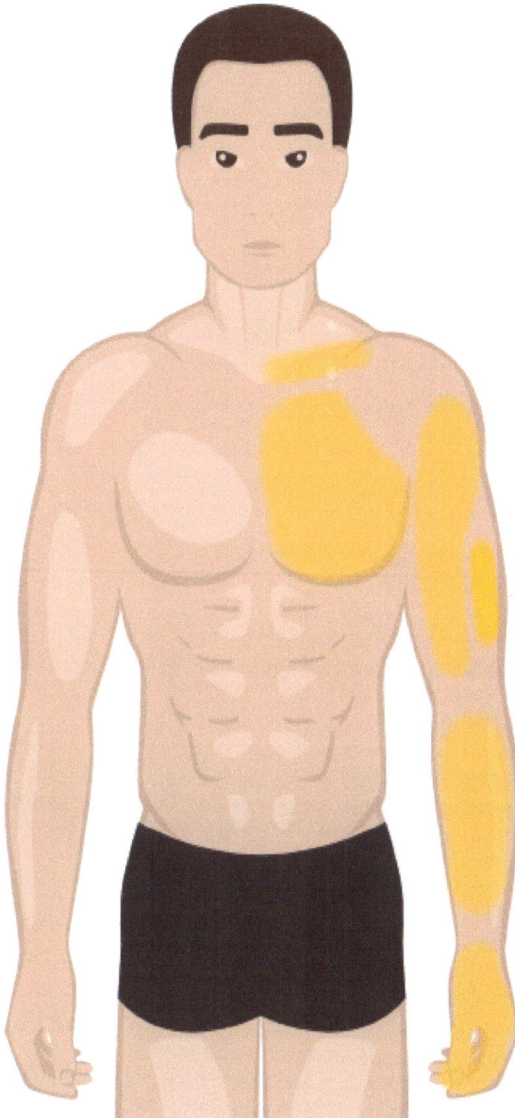

15 et 16. Forearms

17. Biceps

18. Biceps brachialis

21. Hand

24. Clavicle

25. Pectoralis major

26. Pectoralis minor

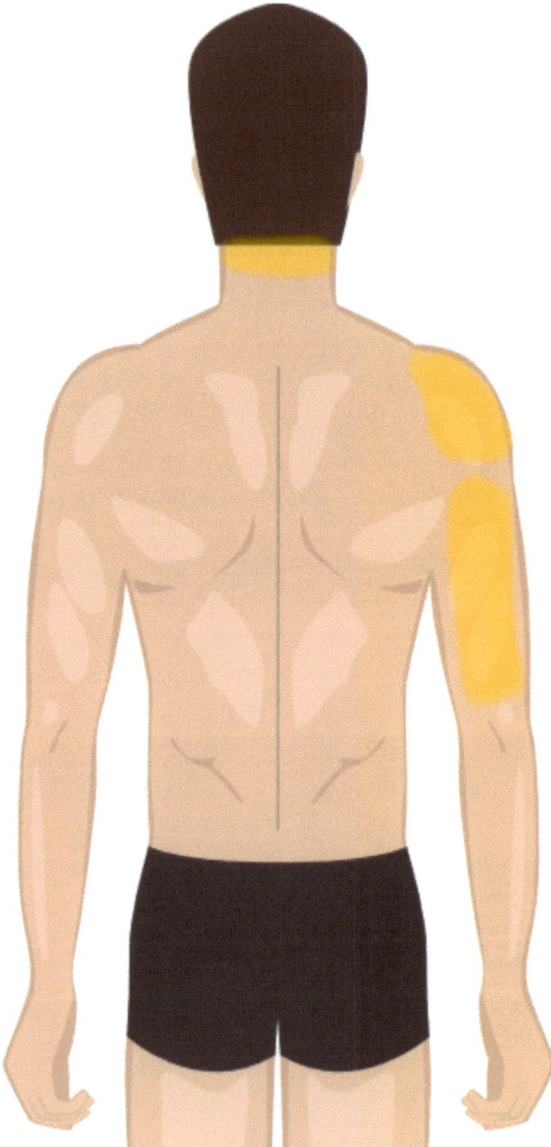

19. Deltoids
23. Occiput
30. Triceps

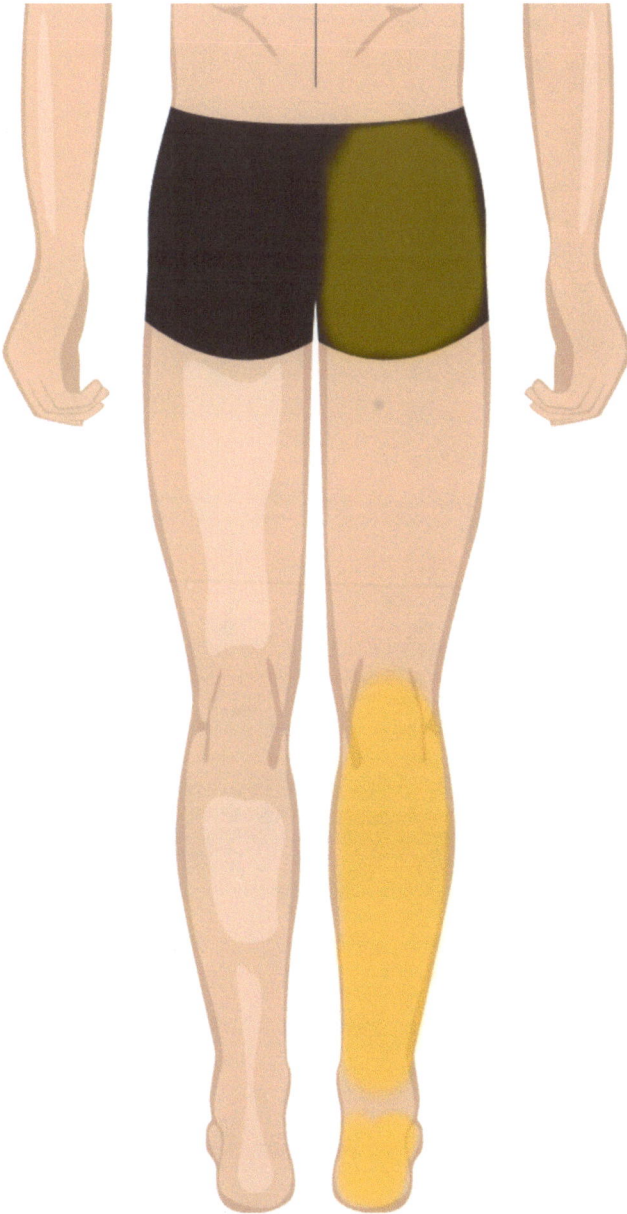

20. Glutes
22. Calf
27. Foot

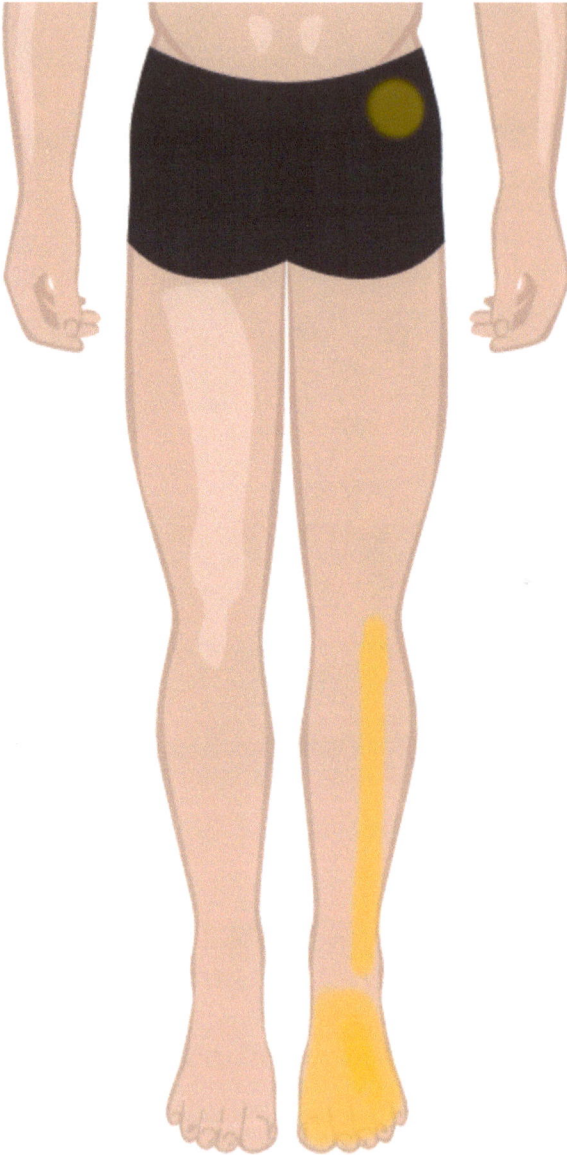

28. Tensor fascia latae (TFL)
29. Tibialis anterior
27. Foot

Muscles to massage

Forearm (Above)

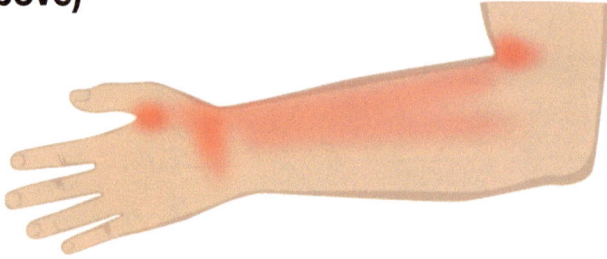

You can relax the top and the bottom areas. Take all your time to explore; it can take some time before the sore spots appear. This body part is often used and, therefore, might require more time before it can relax.

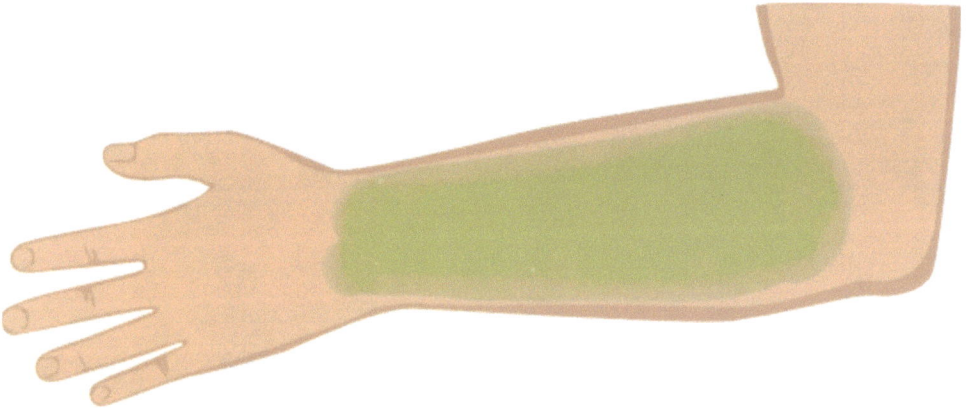

Above: Aim between the two bones and the middle of the forearm. Do not forget the thicker part closer to the biceps.

ℹ️ Recommended if you use your forearms a lot, such as during training or if you are a climber.

Forearm (under)

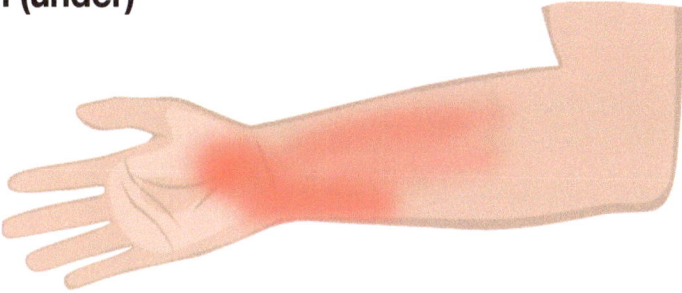

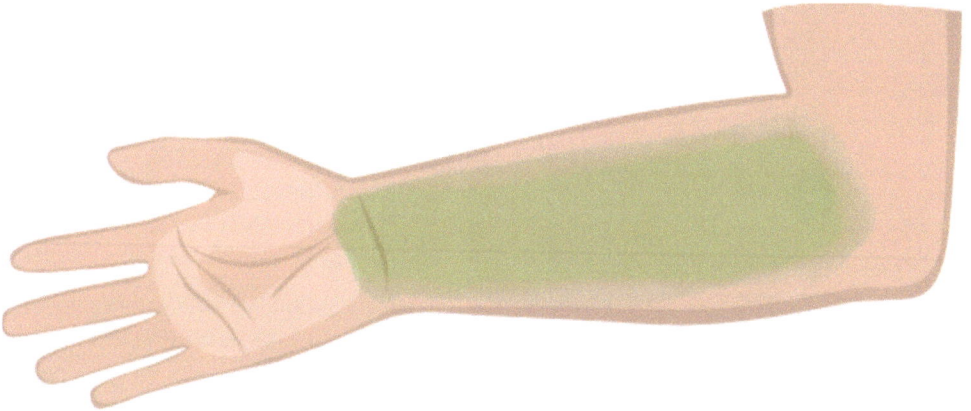

Under: Place your arm on a table, then use the massage gun. You can keep your forearm lifted in the air, but it can prevent the muscles from relaxing fully.

Biceps

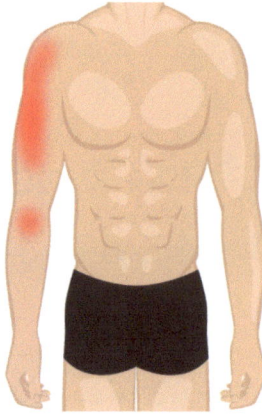

Aim all along the biceps. Often, the most tensed areas are found the furthest from us, close to the elbow.

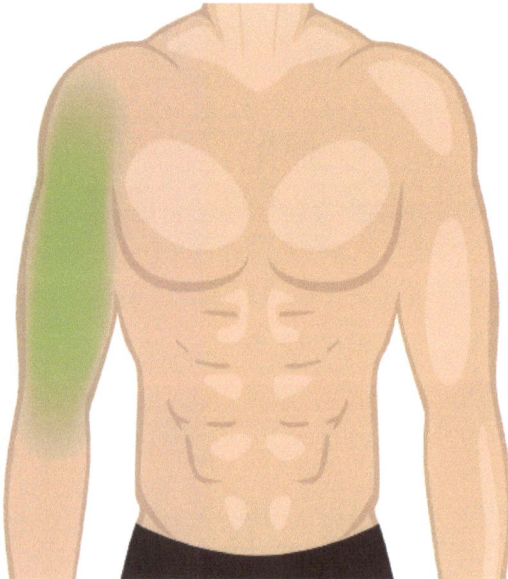

Placement: You can place your arm on a surface or leave it dropping down next to you. It might be better to place it down to keep the muscle more relaxed and less contracted.

Be sure to relax the area that's the furthest from you as it is generally very tensed.

Biceps brachialis

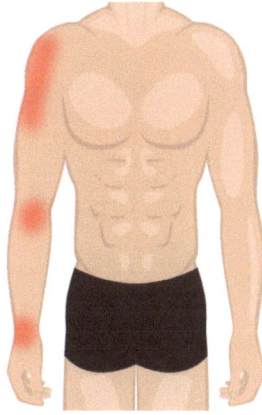

Aim to relax the whole length of your arm, between the biceps and triceps.
You may feel more tension close to the elbow.

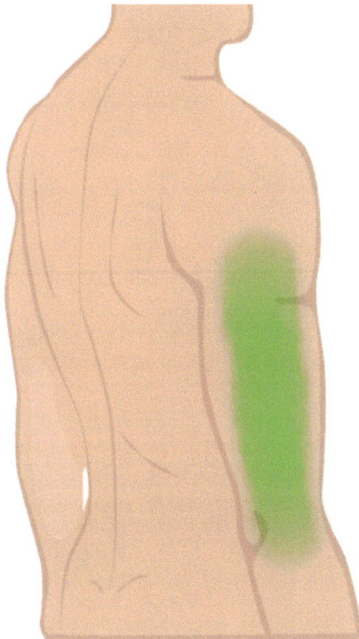

Placement: You can place your arm on a surface or leave it dropping down next to you. It might be better to place it down to keep the muscle more relaxed and less contracted.

ⓘ Be sure to keep the forearm and the arm relaxed and to keep your elbows down.

Deltoids

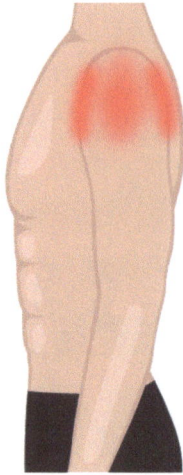

Keep your hand relaxed while you massage the muscle. Aim for the front, the side, and the back of the shoulder to correctly relax the different parts of the deltoids.

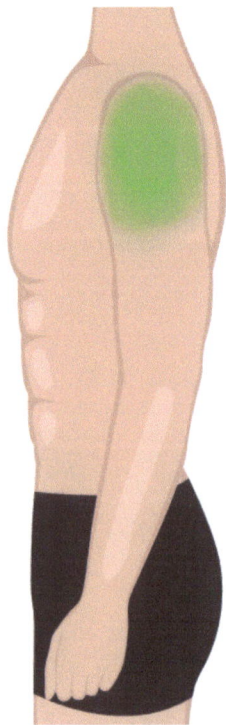

Glutes

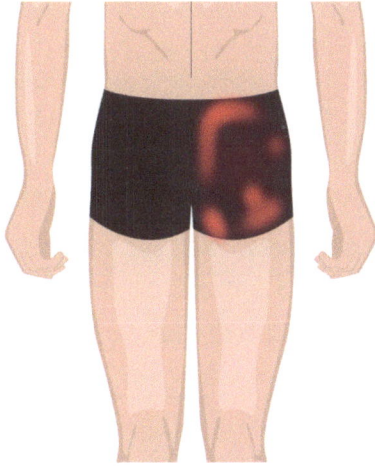

Lay down and turn your hips towards one side to target the sore spots with micromovements such as back and forth or small rotations over the whole muscle. Repeat on the other side.

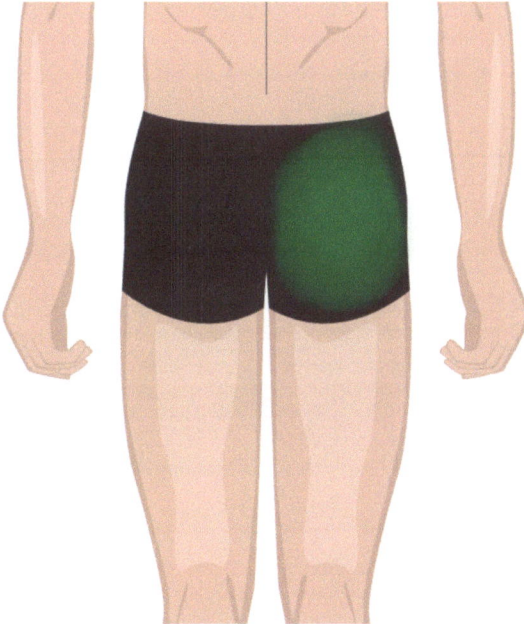

The sore areas are generally along the inner edge of the bone behind the glutes before the groove between the buttocks.

Hand

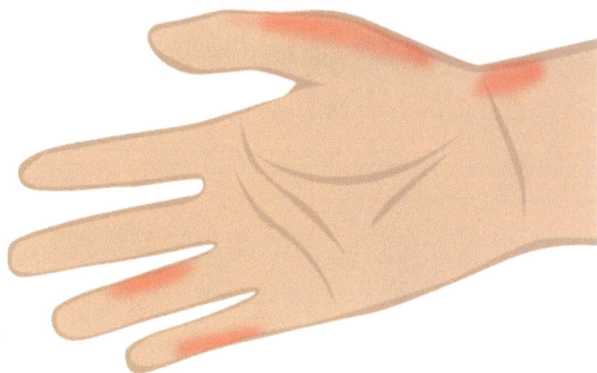

With the gun, relax your palm. It is also possible to massage above and below your wrist.

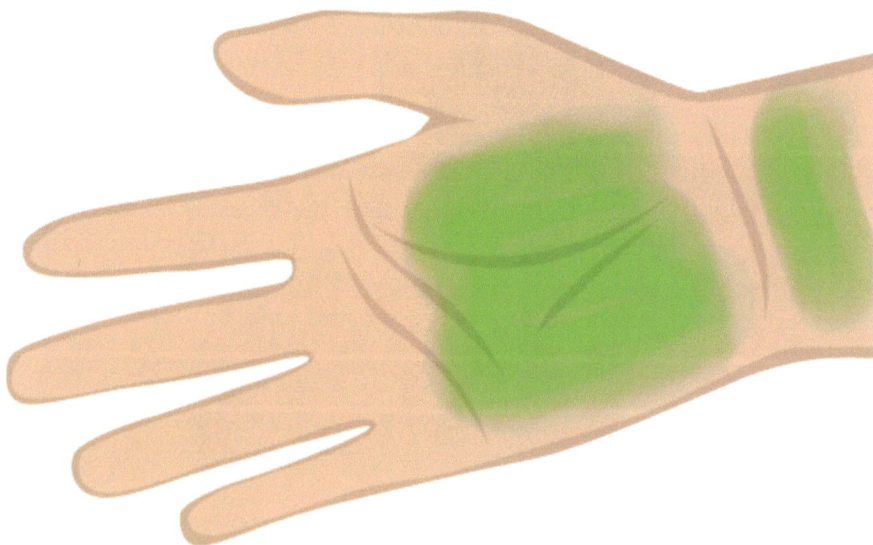

Calf

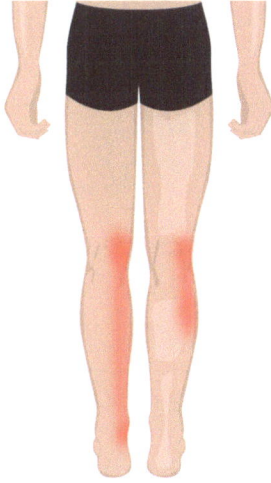

Do back and forth movements and microrotations all along the muscle's length.

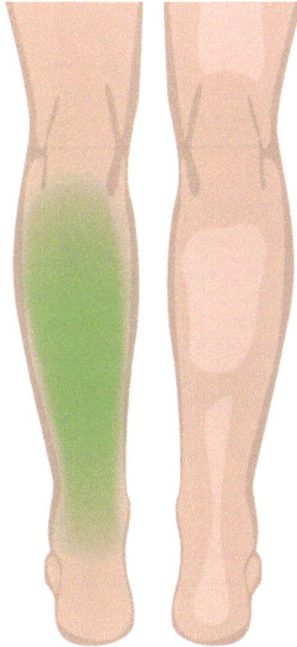

Placement: By sitting down, you can place your calf onto your other leg so that you can have easier access to it.

Occiput

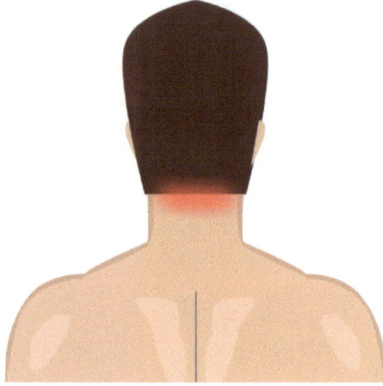

We do not recommend that you use the gun too close to your occipital region as it could make you feel dizzy.

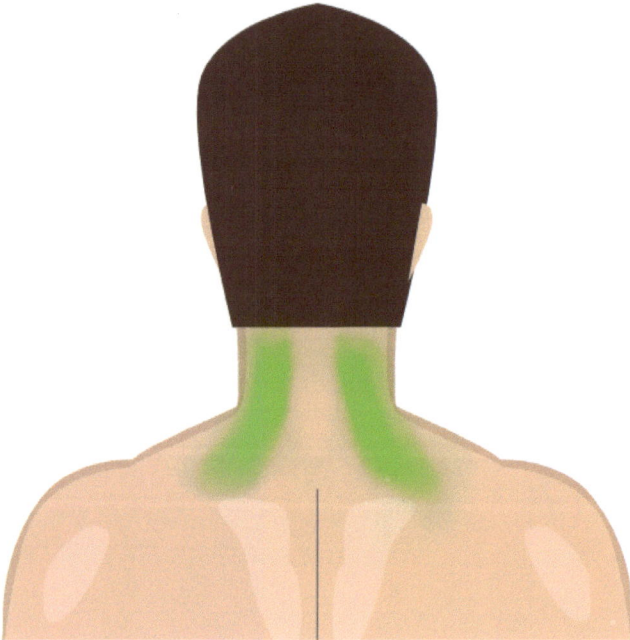

Clavicle

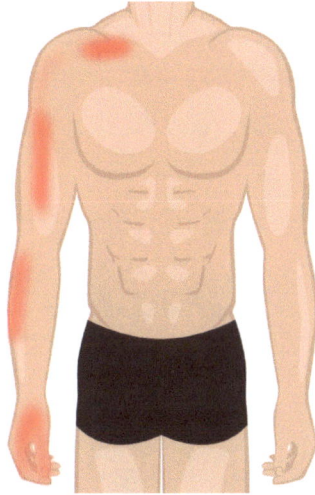

Aim for the part just above the pectoral muscle. The area is situated just below the clavicle and runs for its whole length.

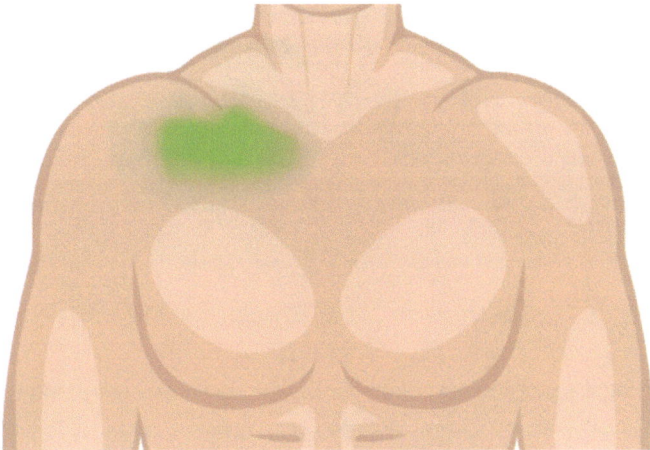

Remember to keep your elbows down and your forearms relaxed.

Pectoralis major

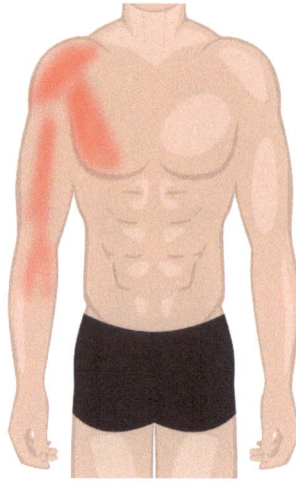

Use the hand on the opposite side to hold the massage gun. You will find the area you need to target close to the muscle's extremities. Be sure to relax the thicker part by accessing it via your side through the armpit.

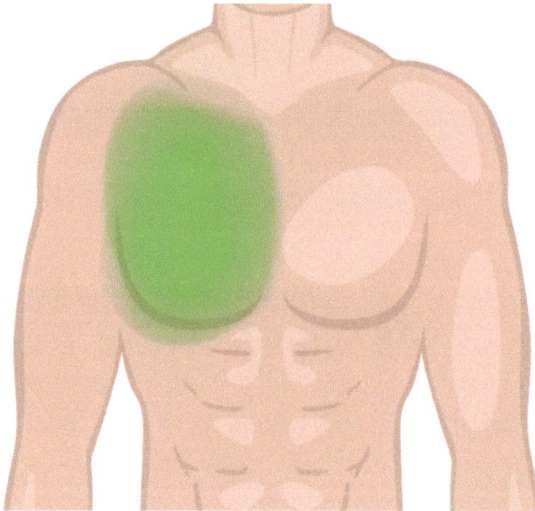

Placement: Varying the position of your arms allows you to roll different parts of the muscle. To start, keep your arm down, then, you can lay it down or position it at different angles.

Make sure to keep your hand and your arms relaxed during your self-massage.

Pectoralis minor

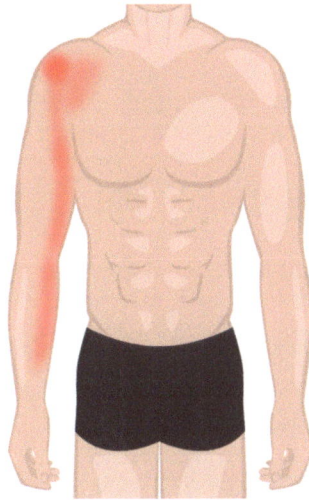

Relax the middle of your torso and toward the sides. You can aim at a specific area if you feel it is necessary by looking at the image. It could feel different when you are massaging directly over the muscle.

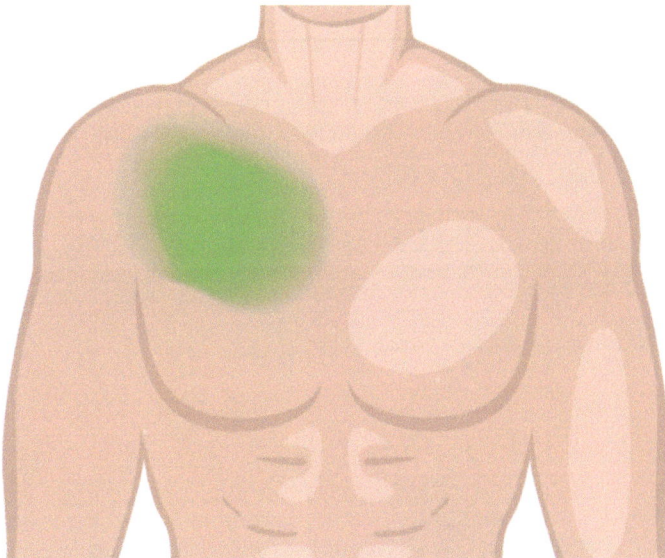

Be sure to keep your hand and your arms relaxed during your self-massage.

Foot

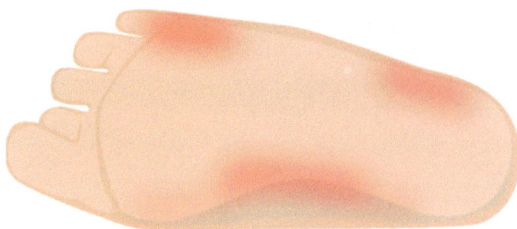

You can relax the middle of the foot, the interior, the exterior part of the arches, the area below your toes, the whole length of the exterior of the foot and your heel. Do small back and forth movements as well as small rotations and stay static on sore spots. You can also relax the top of the foot and its sides.

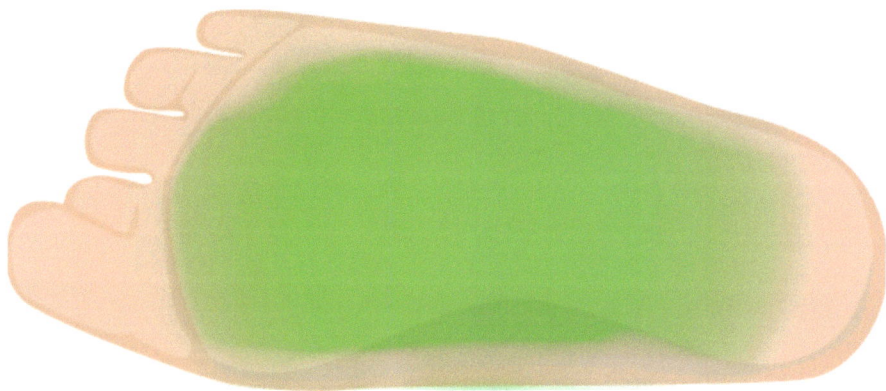

Tensor fascia latae (TFL)

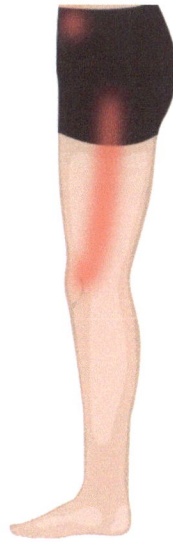

You can release its tensions with the massage gun by aiming it precisely at the areas shown in the image.

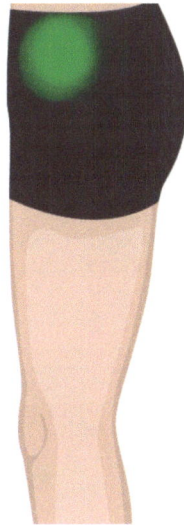

Placement: Find the area between the pointy bone in the front of your hip and the head of the leg's bone. To find it, place your hand along the side of your hip and move the leg; you will find the head of the bone. Then, find the space between both of those two places.

ℹ️ It can be pretty sore or even ticklish.

Tibialis anterior

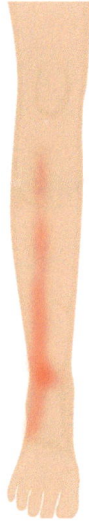

Relax the length of your tibia: the exterior part and close to the middle of the bone. Do back and forth movements as well as small rotations and static pressure points.

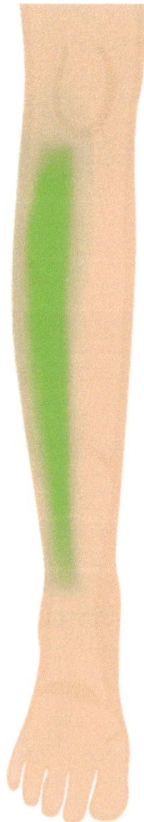

Triceps

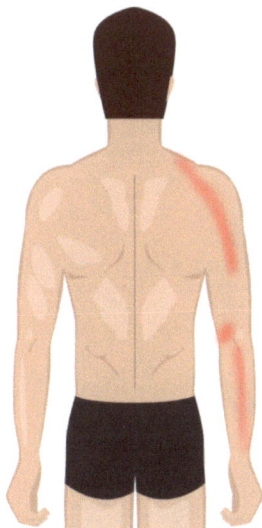

You can use the massage gun to relax the whole muscle. Turn your arm towards the inside of the armpit to reach the back of the muscle more efficiently.

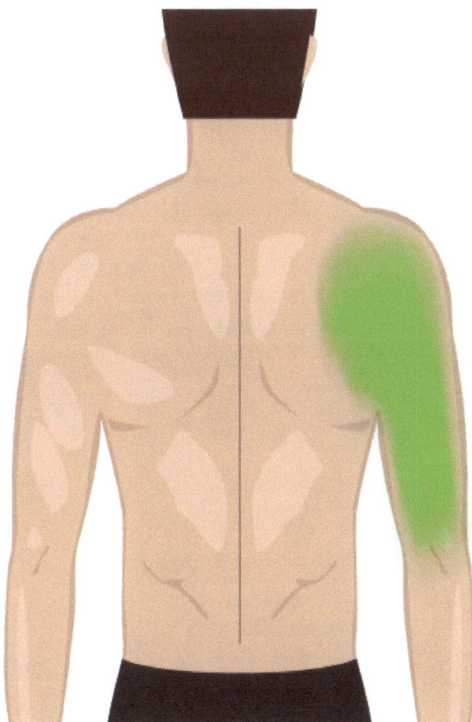

Relaxing your muscles

Our muscles and the tools to relax them

Use the right tool for the right muscle with this table, but do not hesitate to explore them all.

Muscles	Ball	Foam roller	Exercises	Massage gun
Adductors		▯		✓
Biceps	🎾		🧘	✓
Biceps brachialis	🎾		🧘	✓
Calf	🎾	▯		✓
Clavicle	🎾			✓
Deltoid	🎾			✓
Elbow	🎾			✓
Finger extensor			🧘	✓
Finger flexor			🧘	✓

Our muscles and the tools to relax them (continued)

Muscles	Ball	Foam roller	Exercises	Massage gun
Foot	🎾			✓
Forearm	🎾		🧘	✓
Glutes	🎾	▯	🧘	✓
Hand	🎾			✓
Hamstring		▯	🧘	✓
Levator scapulae	🎾		🧘	
Neck	🎾			
Occiput	🎾			
Pectoralis major	🎾		🧘	✓
Pectoralis minor	🎾	▯	🧘	✓

Our muscles and the tools to relax them (continued)

Muscles	Ball	Foam roller	Exercises	Massage gun
Psoas			🧘	
Quadriceps		▯	🧘	✓
Quadriceps lateralis		▯	🧘	✓
Rhomboid	🎾			
Rotator cuff	🎾		🧘	✓
Spinalis		▯	🧘	
Subscapularis			🧘	
Tensor fasciae latae (TFL)	🎾			✓
Tibialis anterior	🎾			✓
Triceps	🎾		🧘	✓

Types of heads

Which head for which need

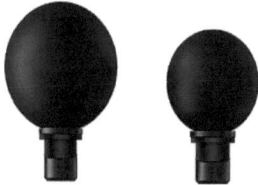

Wide area

A ball that relaxes a wide area and the first layer of the muscles. It's also the most frequent used head.

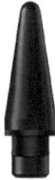

Precision

Some heads are used to target specific areas.

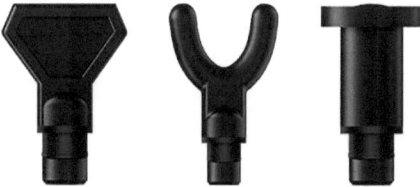

Other types

There is a large variation of heads that are available and that might be different between each brands.

Choosing
the right tool

Common tools for self-massaging

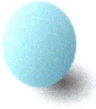

Massage ball

You can use the ball for spots that require precision and for your arms, forearms, and pectorals muscles.

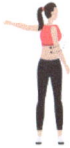

Exercises

The exercises can be helpful for someone who seems really tense and has a hard time relaxing his/her muscles with a self-massage.

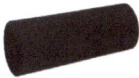

Foam roller

You can effectively use the roller for the largest muscles, such as the legs, the glutes, and the hamstrings. You can also use it to relax your back.

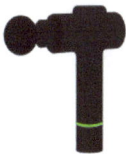

Massage gun

This tool is recommended when you feel your skin is tight, a sore muscle, or you feel your mobility is reduced. It is, however, unable to reach the deepest tensions.

Complete your collection

Also available in this collection

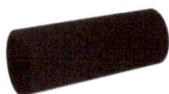

Foam roller
https://massoguide.com/u0jm

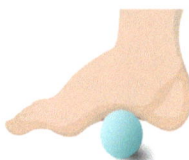

Massage ball
https://massoguide.com/i09r

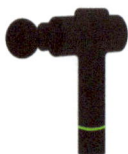

Massage gun
https://massoguide.com/qn8v

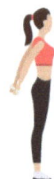

Exercises
https://massoguide.com/5e35

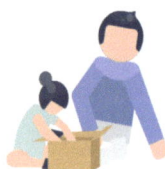

Bad postures
https://massoguide.com/i2yb

Specialized guides for massage therapists

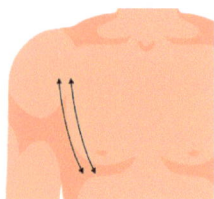

Techniques for good pressure:
Thinking differently
https://massoguide.com/4jax

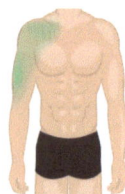

Massage techniques to relieve muscle tension
https://massoguide.com/azoc

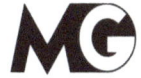

Find your tool

Use the opinions of massage experts on the different self-massage products available.

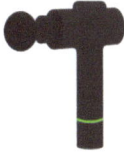

Massage gun

- Batteries
- Accessories

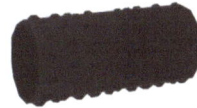

Foam roller

- Lengths
- Surfaces

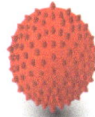

Massage ball

- Sizes
- Surfaces

Help us by sharing your feedback on this guide:

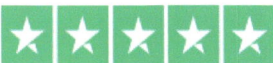

Please! Leave a testimonial

massoguide.com/pwz9

Share on
Facebook!

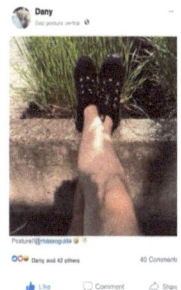

Thanks

These books would not have been possible without the continued support of my entourage and my clients.

A particular thanks is warranted for the exceptional contribution of Christiane Nathalie Geillon. Her help and her friendship were essential in the creation of these books.

About the author

Maxime Marois, a massage therapist, began studying massage therapy after a work injury that required him to seek the help of a physiotherapist. After multiple months of treatment, an interest in understanding the sources of his tensions and his aches developed. It rapidly evolved into a desire to be able to help himself in between the physio visits. This led him to begin a massage course.

This interest in understanding the source of the different issues and the multiple ways to reduce or remove them stayed with him during his career. In noticing the different tensions that his clients would talk to him about, he began to find links between the different tensions and the client's postures. To help his clients in between their massage appointments, he began offering them self-massage advice that would produce quick results.

This knowledge helped him associate the most tensed or sore muscles to the best tools to relax them as well as the most useful self-massage methods and offer this knowledge to the greater public so that they too can benefit and ease their tensions.

www.ingramcontent.com/pod-product-compliance
Lightning Source LLC
Chambersburg PA
CBHW040933030426

42336CB00006B/67